Juice Me! A Complete Juicing Guide for Healthy People

How Juicing Can Help Heal Your Body

By: Stacia G. Browne

9781631871740

I0413956

Publisher's Notes

Disclaimer – Speedy Publishing, LLC

This publication is intended to provide helpful and informative material. It is not intended to diagnose, treat, cure, or prevent any health problem or condition, nor is intended to replace the advice of a physician. No action should be taken solely on the contents of this book. Always consult your physician or qualified healthcare professional on any matters regarding your health and before adopting any suggestions in this book or drawing inferences from it.

The author and publisher specifically disclaim all responsibility for any liability, loss or risk, personal or otherwise, which is incurred as a consequence, directly or indirectly, from the use or application of any contents of this book.

Any and all product names referenced within this book are the trademarks of their respective owners. None of these owners have sponsored, authorized, endorsed, or approved this book.

Always read all information provided by the manufacturers' product labels before using their products. The author and publisher are not responsible for claims made by manufacturers.

This book was originally printed before 2014. This is an adapted reprint by Speedy Publishing LLC with newly updated content designed to help readers with much more accurate and timely information and data.

Speedy Publishing, LLC©2014

40 E. Main Street #1156

Newark, Delaware

19711

Contact Us: 1-888-248-4521

Website: http://www.speedypublishing.com

REPRINTED Paperback Edition: ISBN: 9781631871740

Manufactured in the United States of America

Stacia G. Browne

DEDICATION

For the love of juice, this book is made purely for the intention of sharing my insights about the benefits of juicing. There is power in juice and for that; I would like to share with you that you can beat this lifestyle illnesses of today, and be a better you, inside and out.

TABLE OF CONTENTS

INTRODUCTION

So how do we sustain a healthy body? Generally, we can keep our body in good shape when we feed it with the right nutrition and at the same time we do regular exercise. Physical exercise is known to be very effective in keeping our body working properly. This is because a good exercise can strengthen the immune system which is responsible in defending our body against any diseases. Furthermore, it can also improve our body's digestion, blood circulation and musculoskeletal function.

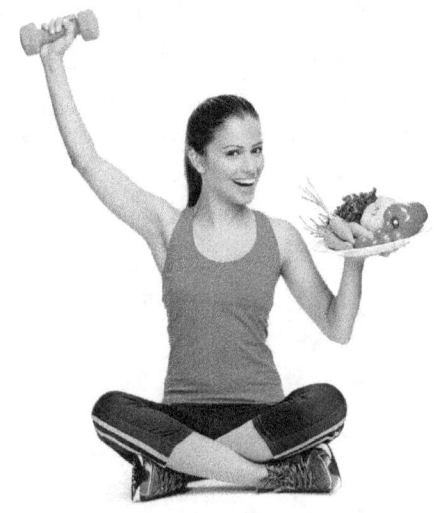

The Basics

Another way of keeping our body healthy is to allow it to have full rest. Through the night, our body is working to repair and maintain body parts that are not functioning well. Therefore, depriving ourselves of sleep will cause us to feel weak and eventually feel fatigued. On the other hand, when we are fully rested our body can easily repair cells and gain enough strength for the next day.

Furthermore, when our body is consistently healthy, we can handle stress easily and we will become more resilient to any infection. In addition, a well maintained body can effectively fight back chronic diseases such as high blood pressure, heart disease, diabetes, cancer and many more. More than that, these diseases can be prevented when we are maintaining a healthy body through exercise and proper nutrition.

On the other hand, staying fit also means keeping a good body build. The more time we spend exercising, the more calories we burn. Based on studies, when we exercise for at least 30 minutes daily, our food intake will be reduced from high to average. This also means that our calorie intake will be balanced, which in result will give us a healthy and controlled weight.

CHAPTER 1- ALL ABOUT NATURAL AND ORGANIC FOODS

Over the years there has been confusion concerning natural and organic foods. Today we will talk about how these two differ from each other. Many people cannot differentiate natural foods from organic, maybe because of how it is labeled and marketed. However, if we study deeper, there is in fact a major distinction between the two.

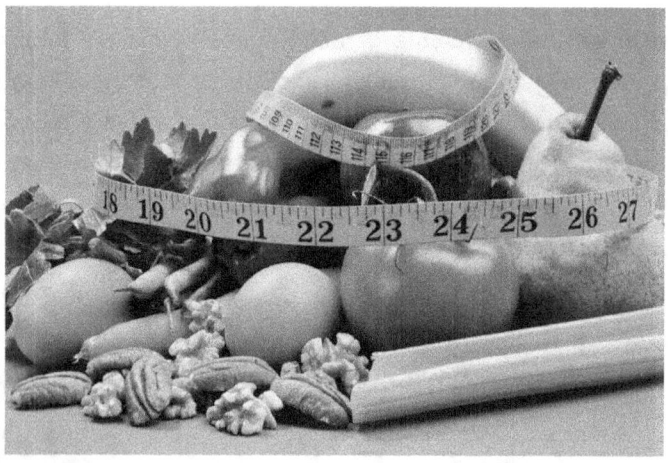

Know the Facts

Organic food is defined as all foods that are grown in the absence of pesticides, fertilizers, irradiation, growth hormones, antibiotics and genetic engineering. Furthermore, it is the product of organic farming where the system used in growing foods enhances biodiversity, soil biological activity and biological cycles. Natural foods, on the other hand, are the foods that are prepared with little or no preservatives as well as chemical additives that are usually present in other processed products.

While it is true that organic foods will lessen the chemicals and pesticides that you get from chemically processed foods, it doesn't mean that you get more health benefits out of it because even non- organic foods are still within safety levels and therefore organic foods are not necessarily more nutritious. The reason why other people choose organic foods over traditional is because it tastes better, but in terms of health, there is not much of a difference.

Furthermore, whether or not the food is organic, the chance of bacterial contamination in food is still uncontrollable. On the other hand, there are other benefits of natural and organic foods which basically include better taste as it has better firmness and texture.

CHAPTER 2- HOW TO SELECT THE RIGHT CARBOHYDRATES

Dietary carbohydrates, also known as saccharine have actual sugars and starches that are responsible in providing energy to humans, animals and even plants. Carbs in a real sense have advantages and disadvantages, especially since right now food production has dramatically changed as well as how food is consumed.

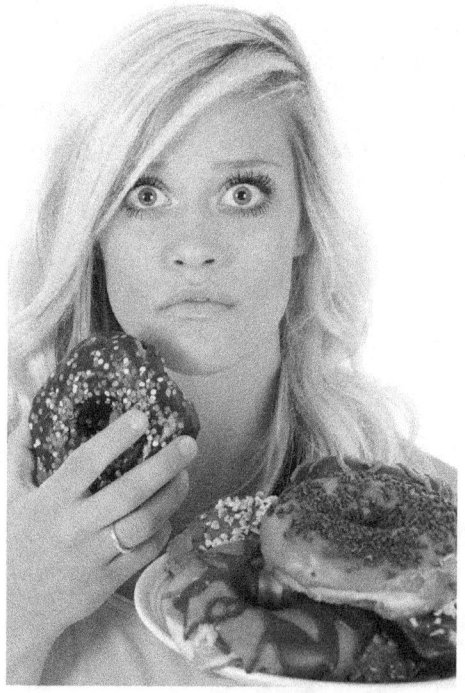

Proper Selection

Carbs have two types, monosaccharides and polysaccharides. Monosaccharides can be easily digested and absorbed by the body.

It is normally obtained in fruits and specific dairy products. Other sources of simple carbohydrates are pastas, white bread and white sugar.

Polysaccharides on the other hand, take a longer period of time to be digested and absorbed by the body. It is normally found in vegetables, legumes, whole grain breads, brown rice and the like. Basically, unrefined grains are a good sources of complex carbs compared to refined grains, this is because the filtering process generally removes the fiber and nutrients present in grains. Therefore, eating unrefined grain products will give you lasting energy.

While carbs are essential in the body, we must make sure that we are picking the right carbs to consume. To do that, we need to understand carbs even better and know how to use them to our advantage. The catch is, we need to eat the right carbs that our body needs in order for us to sustain the right energy.

It is recommended by the experts that for an adult's dietary energy, 40 to 65% percent of it must come from carbs and around 10% of it should be simple carbs. Too many cravings of high-glycemic foods will not only make us fat, but also increases the risk of acquiring diabetes.

Talking about diabetes and weight problems, cutting all carbs in your diet is definitely not the solution. Carbohydrates are very important in providing our body with enough nutrients, vitamins and soluble fiber that is good in maintaining healthy sugar and cholesterol levels.

So how do we choose the right carbs? Here's how. Switch from low- glycemic foods and reduce calorie intake to at most 250-500 calories per day. Moreover, allow yourself to consume 20g to 35g of fiber in a day. One of the best sources of fiber is whole grain foods.

Protein is known as very low in carbs. Consume foods that are lean on protein such as non-fat dairy products, skinless poultry, tofu, legumes and fish. On the other hand, you must avoid foods that are high in saturated fats like pork, high-fat dairy products and beef.

Chapter 3- How to Select the Right Fats

We are perfectly created; therefore even fats have an important role to play. Having said this let me describe fat first. Fat stores energy while it shields our vital organs. It is also known as the passage system of fat-soluble vitamins. Basically, we need it in our body, but only in moderation. Eating fat in large amounts will make us grow heavier and will increase the chance of reaching the level of obesity.

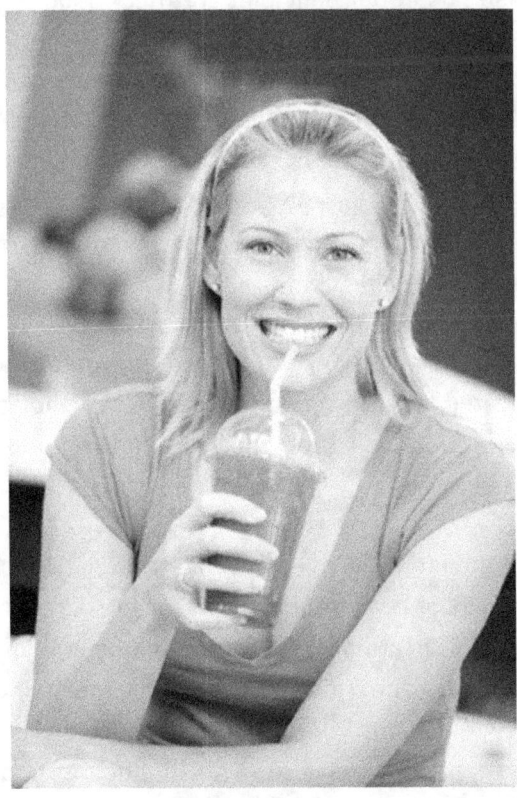

Get the Right Stuff

To stay in the health scope, we must only consume at most 55 to 60 grams of fats per day. There are several types of fat and they are categorized into two broad categories which are, "The bad fats" and "The good fats". Each type has different effects on your health.

The bad fats are identified as Trans fat and Saturated fat. When vegetable oil undergoes a certain process called hydrogenation, trans fat in form. This process causes the oil to harden; as a result hard fats are produced. Moreover, trans fat increases bad cholesterol and decreases good cholesterol levels, this condition increases the risk of having heart disease. The most common sources of bad fats in our daily diet are fried food, cakes, pastries, cookies and the like.

Saturated fat works in the same way with trans fat. It increases bad cholesterol levels that cause heart diseases. Some of the identified sources of saturated fat are fatty meat, margarine, dairy products that contain high fat and other food prepared with coconut milk and palm-based vegetable oil.

On the other hand, the two good fats are polyunsaturated fat and monounsaturated fat. These two reduce the bad cholesterol in the body which in effect will keep the body healthy and away from chronic diseases.

Polyunsaturated fat reduces the dangers of blood clotting and decreases the risk of heart problems. Its major sources are the food rich in omega-3 like sardines, mackerel, salmon and long tail shad. Other sources are canola oil, walnuts, sunflower oil, soybean oil and the like. A Monounsaturated fat also reduces bad cholesterol in the body. The foods that are rich in monounsaturated fat are peanut oils, nuts, canola oil and olive oil.

Apparently, it is easier to exceed fats consumption than to stay in average. But now that you already know the types of fats and their benefits, always choose the good over the bad. Also, strive to consume fats in moderation as even good fats when taken excessively can be harmful to your health.

CHAPTER 4- USING JUICING FOR BETTER PHYSICAL HEALTH

There is no doubt that eating vegetables will make you healthy. The question is will drinking vegetable juices give out equally healthy benefits? Or will it give more? I know you want to know the truth about juicing, that's why you are reading this. To give you this satisfaction, read on and learn more.

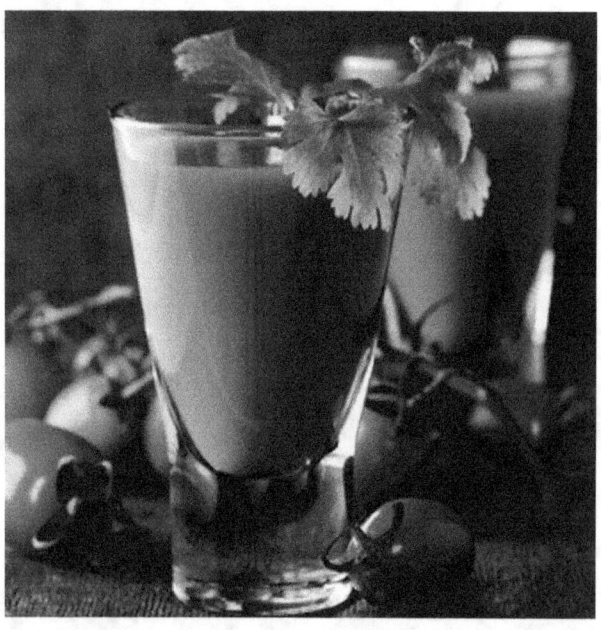

Juicing will allow you to consume more vitamins and antioxidants for an obvious reason; you can consume more vegetables when it is in liquid form compared when you eat vegetables in solid form. Studies show that drinking juice of raw vegetables helps fight back chronic diseases such as immune disorders, high blood pressure, diabetes, cancers, skin diseases and many others.

Furthermore, drinking raw vegetable juices are very good for your digestion because your digestive system uses less energy to digest and liquefy food. Thus, it can rest more. Although you will not be able to benefit much on fiber, you will surely be delighted with the benefits that a live enzyme can give knowing that juicing will preserve the enzymes since the food is uncooked.

Then again, we need to understand that juices are not created the same except when done freshly. For bottled juices, make sure to read the labels because highly concentrated fruit juices can significantly increase blood sugar levels, aside from the fact that it has less nutritional value since it undergone artificial process.

When preparing homemade juices, it should be noted that it is very important to consume the juice product as soon as it is ready as letting it sit will only encourage the growth of pathogens and they also tend to break down faster when exposed to air, thus effectively losing a lot of its originally touted value.

It should also be noted that although consuming juices as a regular habit, limiting the juicing to only fresh fruits, would not be a very good idea as a lot of fruits have a naturally high sugar content and are not so high in fiber, thus causing the negative build up of sugar levers in the body system. This may lead to diabetes and weight gain issues. A better alternative would be to combine complimenting fruits and vegetables together to form one delicious concoction that is both tasty and healthy. Accompanying this with a healthy fat and lean protein diet is also an added advantage.

It is best to prepare fruit and vegetable juices by yourself to ensure optimum benefits. To enjoy it more, you can try combining a few types of fruits and veggies while you experiment until you find your favorites. Nevertheless, you can try some popular mixes such as

Juice Me!
blending leafy vegetable like spinach and cucumber, mixed with apple or carrot to add some sweet taste.

CHAPTER 5- ADVANTAGES OF HEALTHY JUICING

As more people indulge in this form of healthy nutritional intake, it is becoming more popular to consume fruits and vegetable through juicing rather than eating these items as a whole and in its original form.

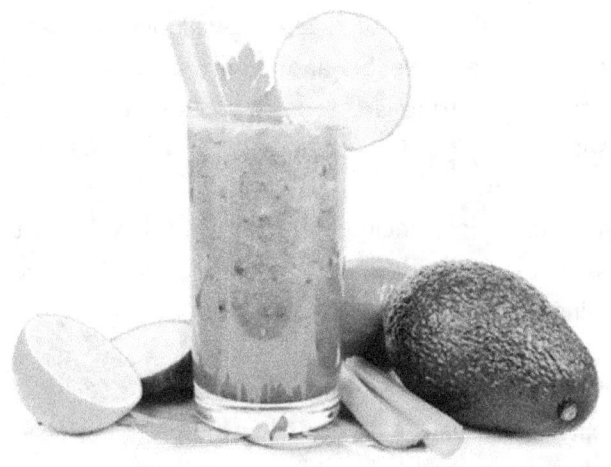

However, scientist and nutritionist are or two minds when it comes to the merits of juicing as opposed to consuming these items whole, although there is yet to be any proven data to merit or advocate either choice over the other.

Advantages

There should however be some knowledge on the matter, before actually making juicing a permanent feature in an individual's lifestyle.

Juice Me!

Studies have shown that juicing is one way of getting all the fruits and vegetable requirements into the body system effectively though, albeit without the positive addition of the fiber needs.

It is arguably a more effective way of getting the nutrients absorbed into the body system without putting undue pressure on the digestive system to break down the fibers.

For those who naturally have a dislike for consuming fruits and vegetable, juicing may present a more acceptable alternative.

There are also a variety of recopies available to make the juicing concoctions more agreeable and even tasty. Juicing combinations of vegetables and fruits are good to include in the recipe sourcing exercise.

Most juicing recipes include the parts of the fruits that would otherwise be discarded in the more conventional way of consuming them.

However, with juicing the inclusion of pits, peelings, seeds and other parts are usually all included in the process since it has been noted that these contain a rich source of vital nutrients which are usually systematically thrown out.

Processed juices usually require some heating process to enhance the shelf life of the product and this can cause the enzymes to be killed. However, with juicing this can be avoided and the enzyme content can be kept intact.

CHAPTER 6- WHEATGRASS-A CLOSER LOOK

Wheatgrass step-ups the red blood-cell count and brings down blood pressure. It likewise cleans the blood, organs and GI tract of debris. Wheatgrass juice taken in each day has been demonstrated to energize metabolism and the body's enzyme systems by enriching the blood. It likewise aids in bringing down blood pressure by dilating the blood pathways throughout the body.

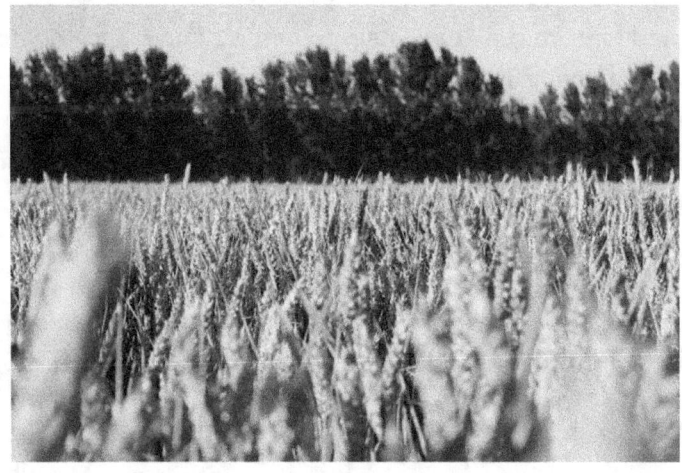

Powerful Friend

Regular ingestion of wheatgrass juice (the most popular way to acquire your daily wheatgrass nutrition boost) energizes the thyroid gland, serving to correct health problems like obesity, indigestion, and a horde of additional complaints.

Wheatgrass juice likewise aids in restoring alkalinity to the blood. The juice's abundance of alkaline minerals helps cut down over-acidity in the blood. It may be utilized to relieve a lot of internal pain, and has been utilized successfully to care for peptic ulcers, ulcerative inflammatory bowel disease, constipation, diarrhea, and additional complaints of the GI tract.

For a lot of people, perhaps the most crucial advantage of wheatgrass is its reputation as a potent detoxifier, offering crucial protection for the liver and blood. The enzymes and amino acids encountered in wheatgrass may protect us from carcinogens like no other food or medicine. It beefs up our cells, detoxifies the liver and bloodstream, and chemically counteracts environmental pollutants.

Wheatgrass in your diet will help to battle tumors and counteract toxins in the body. New studies demonstrate that wheatgrass juice has a potent ability to battle tumors without the common toxicity of drugs that likewise subdue cell-destroying agents. The many active compounds detected in wheat grass juice clean the blood and counteract and digest toxins in our cells.

Scientists have likewise demonstrated that wheatgrass juice holds beneficial enzymes. Whether you've a cut finger you wish to heal or you want to lose some weight... enzymes must do the real work.

The life and powers of the enzymes found naturally in our bodies may be broadened if we help them from the outside by putting in exogenous enzymes, like the ones detected in wheatgrass juice. Don't cook your wheatgrass. We may only garner the advantages of the many enzymes detected in grass by eating it uncooked. Cooking demolishes 100 percent of the enzymes in food.

The nutritive profile of freshly juiced wheatgrass carries remarkable similarity to our own blood. The 2nd important nutritional facet of chlorophyll is its noteworthy similarity to hemoglobin, the compound that transports oxygen in the blood.

Many people are using grass as food and medicine. The reasoning is that since chlorophyll is soluble in fat particles, and fat particles are soaked up directly into the blood via the lymphatic system, that chlorophyll may likewise be soaked up in this way. Put differently, when the "blood" of plants is soaked up in humans, it's transformed into human blood, which channels nutrients to every cell of the body.

CHAPTER 7- WHAT ABOUT SPROUTS?

Sprouts have a lot of useful attributes in respect to human health.

In the 20's, a professor stirred the concept and way of life of Bio-genic nourishment. He classed sprouted seeds and baby greens as the most advantageous foods and advocated that they make up 1/4 of our day- to-day food intake, naming them life-generating Bio-genic foods which he said offer the heaviest support for cell regeneration.

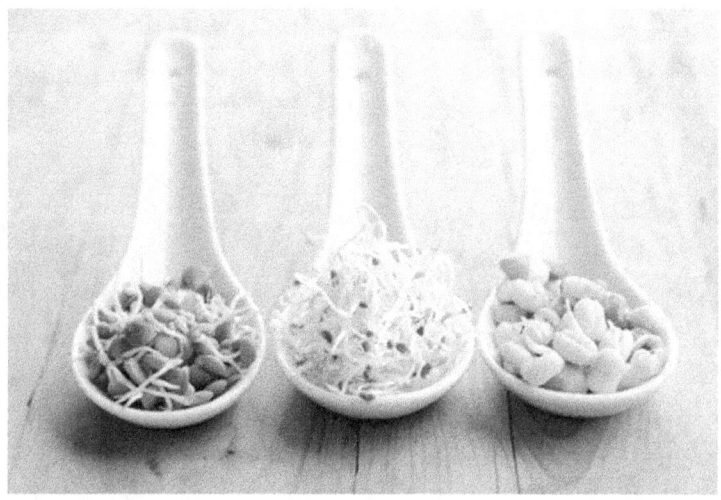

In our day-to-day life, assorted factors transpire to produce free radicals in our bodies. Free radicals are extremely unsound oxygen molecules requiring an electron to stabilize their helter-skelter state.

By sneaking electrons from healthy cells the causal effects of this are the crumbling of life-sustaining biological structures and the modification of DNA and RNA (a procedure known as oxidation).

When this has happened, the impacted cell will only reproduce the changed version. These super foods are a potent origin of antioxidants (minerals, vitamins and enzymes) which help in protecting against this damage.

A fit body is alkaline (i.e. not acidic).Bio-genic foods have an alkalizing impact on the body.

Raw foods bear oxygen and steady consumption of raw bio-genic foods with their abundant oxygen is useful to health.

 It has been found that the growth of cancer cells was originated by a lack of oxygen and these cells, along with viruses and bacteria might not live in alkaline and oxygen rich surroundings.

Bio-genic foods are a great source of crucial fatty acids (the normal western diet is commonly deficient in these) which play a major role in the immune system defenses and are among the highest food sources of fiber.

Once these super foods are grown to the chlorophyll rich 2 leaf stage, it has been demonstrated they were effective in defeating protein-deficiency anemia.

Some women have discovered that daily use of these super foods has yielded relief from hot flushes and sustained hormonal function.

The supply of vitamins (B complex and C) existent in the seeds may be expanded by the sprouting biochemistry over numerous days.

This biochemistry alters the array of minerals in sprouts so that they're in a kelated form which is more simply absorbed in the body.

Juice Me!
It as well denatures protein into the amino acid building blocks so that we may digest them in one-half the time of cooked foods.

CHAPTER 8- GETTING RID OF FAT BY JUICING

Incorporating the juicing exercise into a weight loss diet plan is a very effective way to shed the weight. However, it should be noted that the juicing process should ideally include both vegetables and fruits as concentrating on only fruits will not be beneficial because most fruits usually have high sugar contents.

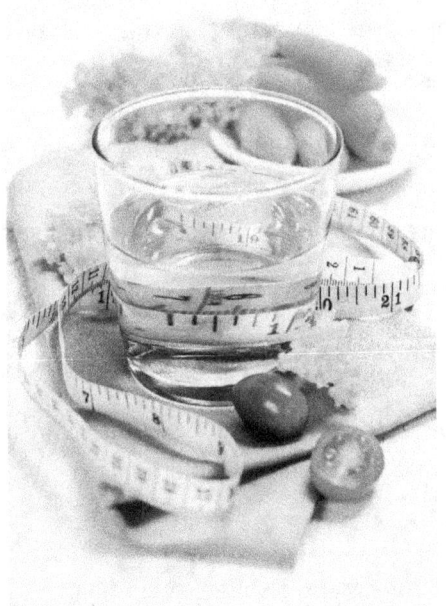

Get the Fat Out

Juicing is also a good ingredient for any detoxifying exercise and it can be used as a meal replacement or when there is a fasting plan in place. If the juicing purpose is meant to detoxify, then it will function to push out all the toxins and fats that have accumulated over time in the body system.

These juices will work as cleansing agents which would be an ideal substitute for a heavy unhealthy meal. Juicing will also be a more healthy and realistic way to lose weight.

Most juicing recipes that are designed for weight loss are very nutritious and satisfying to ensure the individual does not have to resort to supplementing it with other food items due to hunger pangs.

They also usually include ingredients that are specifically part of the combination of the characteristics of sweeping away the toxins and fats.

It is also recommended to ensure that all the ingredients used in the juicing recipes are fresh produce and it should all be cleaned thoroughly before actually commencing the juicing exercise.

The following are some recipes that would serve well in the quest to juicing the fat away:

Apple berry fiber – the apples are excellent cleansing agents while the berries provide the mineral supplements.

Green Pineapple – this concoction is simply refreshing and bursting with goodness and also feels very filling.

Orange pineapple chili – being full of vitamin C, and having enzymes that can dissolve mucus accumulated in the body, it also speeds up the metabolic system.

Gingered pear – a great laxative option and good for digestion.

Stacia G. Browne
Juicing For Kids

Most times it is a struggle for both parents and children when it comes to tackling the issue of eating vegetables and fruits served at meals. However, with the discovery of juicing this problem for most has been eradicated or at the very least decreased to controllable levels.

For The Little Ones

Juicing is a great and fun way to get nutrition into the bodies of growing children to ensure optimal development of their bodies. The trick is to design concoctions that are pleasant to drink and is also refreshing, especially after a strenuous playing session.

However, for younger children it would be advisable to dilute the juices, as the concentrated form may be too much for the underdeveloped body to deal with.

Teenagers and older kids have problems with drinking concentrated juices. Introducing juices to kids should be done in a gradual process with initial stages of diluting.

Choosing fruits that have delectable tastes is much better and less likely to be rejected by the child. Starting out with single juice choices before moving on the combinations is also advised, as this will allow the body system and the child's palate to get used in this introduction into the healthy daily diet plan.

Changing the juices and providing a variety is definitely an attractive feature for children and they would be fascinated with the colors and tastes reflected in the variety.

Juice Me!

Once the favorite juices are identified, serving them as often as possible without boring the child will be beneficial. Using the favorite juice as a base, it may also be possible to add on a little portion of other fruits or vegetables to further enhance the nutrient content of the juice.

Some popular choices may include apple juice, pineapple and carrot juice, orange juice, orange and carrot juice pear juice and apple and grape juice.

Juicing For Anti-aging

Juicing is not the new fad to combat natural aging processes. It makes sense to opt for this healthier and cheaper yet no less effective way of staying off the aging process.

Juicing benefits the body as it provides the combination of all the essential vitamins, minerals, amino acids, essential fatty acids, and enzymes.

These fruits and vegetable that are usually used in the juicing process are also power packed with anti aging and life preserving elements, thus the choice made to incorporate regular juicing exercises would benefit greatly.

The antioxidants and substances that neutralize the free radicals in the system ideally provide the possibility of having well anti aging benefits.

A diet rich with vitamins and minerals is the key factor in fighting against the aging process and one of the most pleasant ways of doing this is through the juicing exercise.

Brightly colored fruits and vegetables are especially beneficial in the anti aging fight. Fruits such as oranges, cherries, tangerines, apples, blueberries, cranberries, melons, bananas, grapes, berries, kiwi, and mangoes are all known for the anti aging properties.

These can be taken in combinations or separately, whichever is suitable for the individual's palate. When it comes to vegetable there is the abundant choice of carrots, squash, red and green cabbages, broccoli, spinach, which are just as beneficial for their anti aging properties too.

Apple carrot detox – 1 apple, 1 slice of ginger, 1 carrot, ½ cup or water. Its excellent properties that create healthy skin and eliminates toxin from the body is the reason this juice is a popular choice for many.

Cholesterol burner – 1 apple, ½ cucumbers, 4 stalks of celery, ½ cup of water. This juice is a good controller of high cholesterol levels in the body system and also helps to fight against upset stomachs, besides the more obvious anti aging properties it carries.

CHAPTER 9- DETOXING BY JUICING

The juicing process is ideal for detoxification of the body system, as it enhances the enzymes, vitamins and mineral absorption which in turn greatly benefit the immune system.

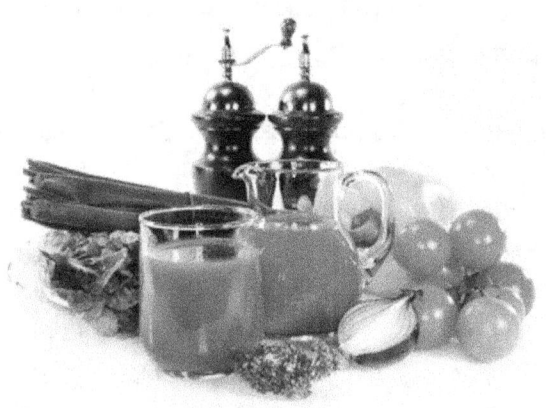

Detox

Juicing organic vegetables and fruits which are rich in nutrients will help to cover the cells in the body with the alkaline juices released from these juicing concoctions whereby acids are released and toxins can be removed through various elimination channels in the body.

The parts of the body that play an important role in filtering such toxins would include the lungs, kidneys, skin and other functions like urination and bowel movements.

The enzymes released from these juices also help the digestive processed where the proteins break down the foods into nutrients and this is an important function as most adults have already used up their natural digestive enzymes by the age of 30.

Therefore the outside aid that the juices provide is definitely beneficial to the digestive process as it is pivotal in the detoxifying regiment the body naturally enlists.

When the body is full of toxins, it is unable to absorb the nutrients that are available in the natural intake of regular foods, thus the need for these added juices to assist in the breakdown of the toxins to cleanse the body and carry the appropriate amount of oxygen and nutrients directly to the cell and tissues.

Some of the ideal ingredients to use in the juicing process for detoxifying would include lettuce, dark green kale, carrots, beet greens, cilantro, parsley, celery sticks, collard greens, endive, spinach, dandelion greens, cabbage both purple and green and lemons.

Some people who practice this detoxifying regiment periodically attest to the fact that they no longer have cravings for sweetened foods and they can keep to a regular and healthy diet without any struggles. This is probably due to the fact that the body is able to function at its optimum because of the detoxifying sessions.

CHAPTER 10- HEALTHY JUICING RECIPES

There are a lot of positive reasons that eventually encourage more people to juicing and this may include the ability to save cash due to the fact that the fruits can be bought in bulk, the definite benefits it can bring to controlling weight gain and shrinking the waistline, creating a fulfilling and healthy diet plan and increasing the energy and vitality levels in an individual.

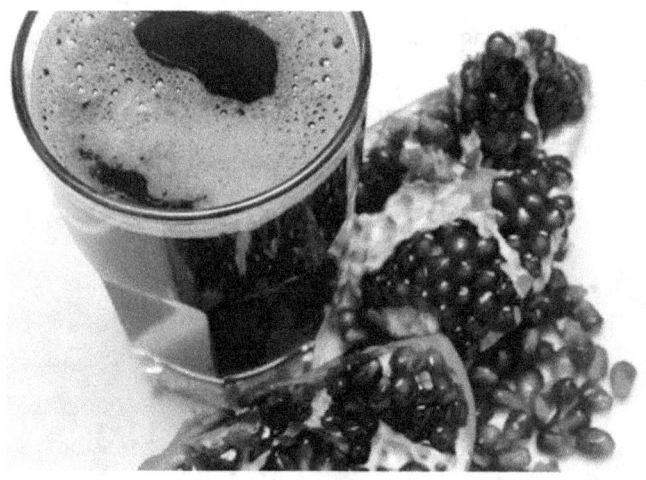

Recipes

The following are some of the more popular juice recipes for the avid juicer:

Lemony Apple – 2 apples, 1 lemon, 1" slice of ginger. This is a healthy remedy for colds as it is rich in flavonoid content. It also has a fresh and tangy taste that is quite invigorating.

Plain O'O. J – 4 medium sized oranges. Remembering to include as much of the white membranes as possible is a good idea as this too is rich in bio-flavonoid. However, in this case it would be a good idea to avoid including the whole peel as it might enhance the sour and raw taste, thus causing the juice to take on a rather unpleasant taste.

Alkaline juice – 1 cup of spinach, ½ cup of cucumber, 2 stalks of celery including the leaves. 3 carrots and ½ an apple. The skin of the dark green cucumber will provide the source of chlorophyll, which is a phytochemical that can help to build up the red blood cells. The cucumbers also contain silica, which is a mineral that is good for the skin.

A Very Berry Medley – 2 cups of strawberries, 2 cups of blueberries and 1.5 cups of raspberries. Berries are a popular choice for juicing due to its quick and easy breakdown process and its simple rinse action. Being a great source of antioxidants such as anthocyanins, flavonoid and ellagic acid, all of which have good anti cancer and anti heart disease benefits.

Pomegranate juice – 5 pomegranates. In this recipe only the seeds are used and the rest of the fruit is discarded. However, some may find better results using a blender as the seed does present a challenge to break down.

CHAPTER 11- WHAT ABOUT ORGANIC FOODS?

At one time found only in health food stores, organic food is today a regular feature at many supermarkets. And that's produced a bit of a quandary in the produce aisle. On the one hand, you've a conventionally grown apple. On the other, you've one that's organic. Both apples are crisp, shiny and red. Both supply vitamins, and fiber, and both are fat free, and have no sodium and cholesterol. Which should you select?

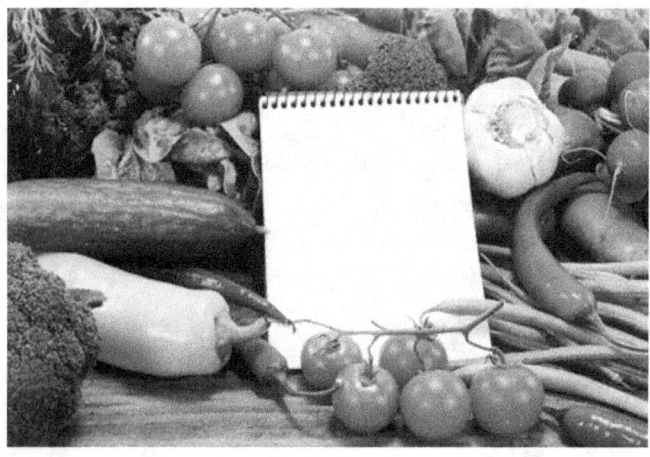

What You Need To Know

Conventionally grown produce commonly costs less; however, is organic food safer or more nutritious? Find the facts before you shop. The word "organic" denotes the way farmers grow and process agricultural products, like fruits, veggies, grains, dairy products and meat.

Stacia G. Browne

Organic agricultural practices are designed to further soil and water conservation and cut down pollution. Farmers who raise organic produce and meat don't utilize conventional techniques to fertilize, contain weeds or prevent livestock disease. For instance, instead of utilizing chemical weed killers, organic farmers might conduct more advanced crop rotations and spread mulch or manure to keep weeds cornered.

The U.S. Department of Agriculture has established an organic certificate program that requires all organic foods to fit strict government standards. These measures, regulates how such foods are raised, handled and processed.

Any product marked as organic must be a Department of Agriculture certified. If a food holds a Department of Agriculture Organic label, it means it's produced and processed according to the Department of Agriculture criteria. The seal is voluntary, but a lot of organic producers utilize it.

Products demonstrated 95 percent or more organic display this Department of Agriculture seal.

Products that are totally organic — like fruits, veggies, eggs or other single-ingredient foods — are marked 100 percent organic and may carry the Department of Agriculture seal.

Foods that have more than one component, like breakfast cereal, may utilize the Department of Agriculture organic seal plus the following wording, contingent on the number of organic ingredients:

100 percent organic. To utilize this phrase, products must be either totally organic or made of all organic components.

Organic. Products have to be at least 95 percent organic to utilize this term.

Products that bear at least 70 percent organic ingredients might state "made with organic ingredients" on the label, but might not utilize the seal. Foods bearing less than 70 percent organic components can't utilize the seal or the word "organic" on their product labels. They may include the organic items in their ingredient list, all the same.

Do 'Organic' and 'Natural' Mean the Same Thing?

Nope, "natural" and "organic" are not exchangeable terms. You might see "natural" and other terms like "all natural," "free-range" or "hormone-free" on food labels. These descriptions have to be truthful, but don't mix them up with the term "organic." Only foods that are raised and processed according to Department of Agriculture organic criteria may be labeled organic.

Conventional growers utilize pesticides to protect their crops from molds, insects and diseases. If farmers spray pesticides, this may leave residue on produce. Some individuals purchase organic food to restrict their exposure to these residues. According to the USDA, organic produce bears significantly fewer pesticide residues than conventional produce. All the same, residues of most products — both organic and inorganic — don't surpass government safety thresholds

A recent study analyzed the past 50 years' worth of scientific articles about the nutrient content of organic and conventional foods. The investigators concluded that organically and conventionally produced foodstuffs are like in their nutrient content. Research in this area is in progress.

CHAPTER 12- THE DANGERS OF UNHEALTHY EATING

A sound diet is associated with infinite advantages, including a bettered immune system, reduced risk for sickness and disease and bettered longevity; when the years of unhealthy eating pile up, these factors might suffer. An unhealthy diet increases one's odds of developing grave conditions like osteoporosis, hypertension and cardiovascular diseases. To preclude such illnesses, consider a balanced, nutrient-rich diet long before symptoms kick in for best results.

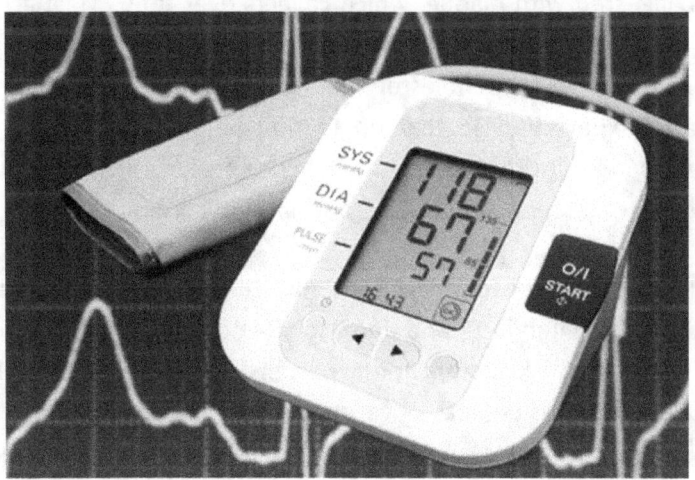

Health Risks

Osteoporosis concerns brittle bones that run a high risk of breaking. Osteoporosis comes along primarily in elderly grownups, frequently as a result of a lifetime of mediocre nutrition. As young grownups, as young as early 20s in the case of adult females, calcium starts to bit by bit deplete from your bones. If you don't eat enough calcium, vitamin D and vitamin C or if your body weight stays dangerously low for long periods of time, your danger for osteoporosis grows dramatically.

To cut down your chances of acquiring osteoporosis, eat an assortment of calcium-rich foods, like low-fat dairy products, calcium-fortified breads, grains, juices and soy milk, spinach, salmon, sardines and tofu on a regular basis. Citrus, tomatoes and strawberries are favorable sources of vitamin C, and you may acquire vitamin D by getting out into the sun daily for short periods. Vitamin D is likewise present in many fortified dairy or soy products.

Hypertension, or high blood pressure, happens when your arteries get congested with plaque, which collects over time. Most arterial plaque is diet-derived and commonly stems from saturated fats, trans fats and dietary cholesterol intake in addition to overeating in general. Experts advise that up to fifty percent of grownups in America are at risk for acquiring hypertension, increasing their odds of stroke, renal failure, heart attack and coronary failure.

Being heavy or obese, consuming too much sodium or too little potassium or vitamin D, and unreasonable consumption of alcohol are significant risk factors for hypertension. To forestall or help reduce hypertension, eat a variety of healthy foods, like fruits, veggies, whole grains and lean protein sources, and cut back on adding sugars, saturated fats and fried foods. Regular physical activity is likewise a means of forestalling hypertension.

Cardiovascular conditions and diseases, like heart disease, arteriosclerosis, congestive heart failure, heart attack and stroke, are grievous, possibly life-threatening diseases that might result from years of unhealthful eating. A healthy diet is one of the most efficient tools you have towards combating heart disease. Foods like saturated fats (found in fatty meats, cheese, butter and eggs) and trans fats (found in shortening, margarine, fried foods and processed snack foods) step-up risk for cardiovascular diseases. Nutrient-rich foods, like fruits, veggies, whole grains, legumes and other lean protein sources, might decrease risk of such diseases. Additionally, at least 2 servings of fatty fish, like salmon, tuna, or mackerel, per week, as they supply the body with omega-3 fatty acids, heart-healthy fats the body needs.

To maintain long-term health and prevent diet-related diseases, stick to a balanced diet, rich in an assortment of nutritious foods.

Wrapping Up

Eating Healthy enables you to better deal with tension! Tension may take its toll on your wellness. That's a fact. Nevertheless, by eating right and taking care of yourself, you may cut back that tension to a manageable level and step-up your productivity and enjoyment of life. By making a list of health priorities and sticking to it, you may earn more, live better and live longer. Your increased productiveness now will pay off huge dividends when the time comes to choose how you wish to live the rest of your life.

You may better the overall quality of your life simply by consuming healthy foods.

It has already been established that juicing is a very healthy exercise to practice. This is also one of the contributing factors that ensure the individual's chances of developing any medical problems are considerably lessened. By lowering the risk of having diseases the juicing habit has proven to be one that everyone should consider for its merits.

Staying Healthy

Juice Me!

There are several very specific combinations that can be used regularly by creating the ideal effects within the body system that allow it to resist any possible occurrences of diseases.

One of which, is drinking a Beetroot combination, as this is said to dramatically reduce the risks of heart disease, strokes, Alzheimer's and dementia.

The bright red juice contains the chemical nitrate, which dramatically reduces blood pressure for almost everyone taking this remedy.

Another juice combination is the one with pomegranate content which is pivotal in lowering cardiovascular risks; however, this should be taken with care as the potassium content is rather high. Tomato juice combinations are also supposed to help lower heart diseases and control diabetic symptoms.

Other benefits of consuming tomato juice would include the resistance to developing chronic diseases like cancer and coronary heart disease. This can be avoided because of the carotenoid content called lycopene which is richly found in tomatoes.

Some of the ingredients that can be used to combat or at least lower the risks of diseases would include broccoli, Brussels sprouts, butter squash, cabbage, Chinese broccoli, kale, spinach, parsley, collard greens, mustards green, chard, beetroot, carrots, cauliflower, cucumber, green pepper, sweet potatoes, lettuce and celery.

Regular combinations of these juices will help to keep the chemical balance in the body system which in turn will allow the body to perform at its prime, thus effectively avoiding any diseases.

CHAPTER 13- RELIEVE STRESS BY JUICING

Almost everyone adult and child alike has experienced bouts of stress at various points in their daily life. For most, this is taken in stride until it is no longer possible to do so, and when this happens it almost always affects the health conditions.

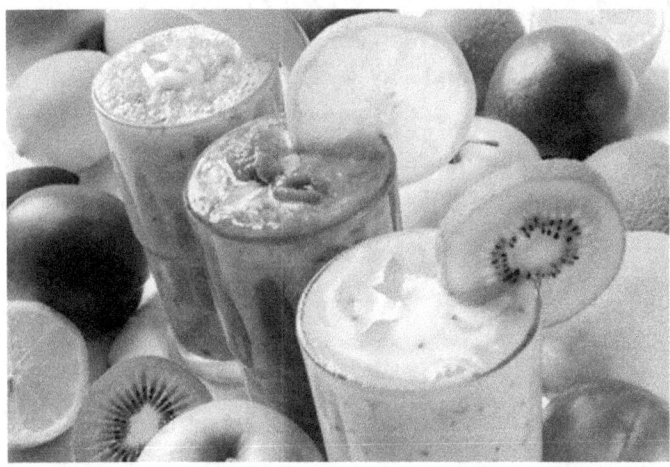

De-stress

Fruit and vegetable juices have long been known for their stress relief and relaxation properties. Therefore taking the time to explore this healthy alternative to popping pills to relieve stress is certainly worth the effort.

Apple, cherry and blueberry ingredients have been known to be good health boosting elements where the flavonoid can facilitate better lung functions and with this optimum breathing position the ideal amounts of oxygen is then able to be circulated well with the body system thus relieving any internal pressures felt when stress levels are high and this eventually helps to lower the stress levels.

These ingredients can also contribute to relaxing the arteries and lowering the risk of cardiovascular diseases which are often caused by stress. Smoothies made from bananas, strawberry, peppermint and lemon can all help to relieve stress and create the relaxing overall body feeling.

When the adrenaline levels increase the body requires more vitamin C and as this cannot be naturally conjured by the human body there is a need to have this supplemented for outside sources, thus the advantage of the aforementioned ingredients.

Bananas would contribute to stress relief properties while the peppermint which contains menthol will have a cooling effect on the body while the others will help in digestion, thus creating an overall effect that will combat any significant presence of stress.

CHAPTER 14- THE ADVANTAGES OF EATING RIGHT FOR A HEALTHY BODY

As we all know, eating the right foods in the right amounts will give us the maximum benefits. However, most of us are not well educated on the right types of food that are needed by our body to function properly. Some of us don't even know when to just stop eating. When we eat the right kind of food we are allowing the body to be properly nourished. Hence, as a result, we will be able to gain health benefits from our healthful efforts.

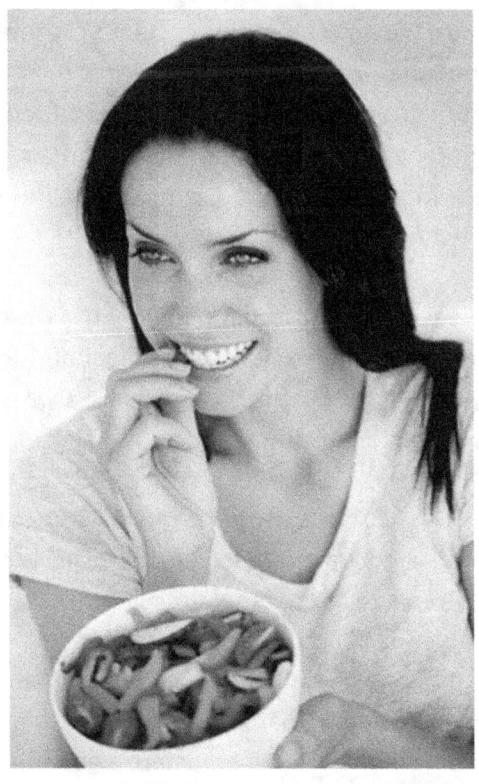

The Rewards

There are several benefits of eating the right food. Below is the list.

1. Maintains a healthy body weight

2. Maintains a normal blood sugar level

3. Reduces the risk of heart attacks

4. Reduces the risk of cancer

5. Improves good blood circulation and maintains stable energy levels

However, despite the above mentioned benefits a lot of people still tend to avoid eating right for the reason that they are under the impression that whether or not they eat good food, there is not much of a difference in their health status. Others tend to avoid eating the right food because they cannot afford to live in such a healthy lifestyle.

It is true that each of us have different needs. Thus, it would be better if we discover and explore more healthful ideas that will best suit us. In general, health professionals always recommend eating the right food for a healthier body.

A healthy diet is composed of protein, fats, carbohydrates, vitamins, minerals and water. These elements need to be taken in proportion to be able to get optimum results.

The good thing about this idea, when you start eating the right foods, there is a possibility that your family and friends will begin to follow. Aside from that, when you start a good habit and strive to really carry on with it, chances are you will become more

Stacia G. Browne

motivated to continue what you are doing. Thus, staying away from unhealthy foods will never be that difficult again.

Maintaining a healthy body and mind really is not that difficult of a task. In reality, part of the hardest part is making the decision to make some changes in your lifestyle. The sooner you can be honest with yourself about the choices you make in your life the sooner you can begin to live healthy. Properly maintaining your body is essential to handling the stresses of everyday life. It is also crucial in maintaining energy levels we need to accomplish our daily tasks.

Chapter 15- Foods to Avoid

I know most of us can relate when I say that there will always be that bad food that we don't want to give up no matter how badly we want to get healthy and fit. What we can do is to identify and be familiar with our usual food intake. We can list down all of those foods we eat and identify the foods that we need to give up or consume in strict moderation.

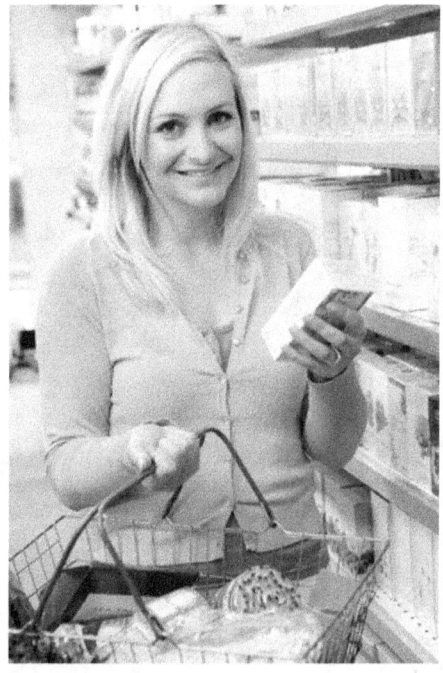

What to Avoid

To guide us through this, we can consider the below guidelines to help us succeed in keeping our body fit. Generally, we should know as to what level we should be avoiding such foods.

Stacia G. Browne

First in the list is red meat. If we want to stay healthy, we need to throw out red meat from our diet as it will not give us any good. It is best that we go for white meat instead. Next would be frozen and processed food. These foods are high in calories and contain preservative chemicals. The majority of us are consuming frozen and processed foods because of the convenience it brings. However, we must pay greater attention to our health than our convenience.

Also, we are well aware that fast foods are not good at all. Kick it out to give way to healthier and tastier foods. Soft drinks are one big temptation. A lot of people are addicted to sodas. If you are one of them now is a high time for you to give up your favorite soda and let your body become chemical and sugar free. When you do that, your body will thank you forever.

Alcoholic drinks are definitely included in the list. It is not bad to drink alcohol when taken in moderation. However, if you want to lose weight while obtaining a healthy body, it is best to just drop the idea of drinking. Normally we can avoid drinking alcohol if we have illnesses that we need to treat; therefore pulling out from alcoholic drinks is definitely possible.

Lastly, when all the aforementioned foods are eliminated in your regime, you can be sure that you will become healthier and leaner. Of course it will not happen in an instant and things will happen gradually. Don't leave off and continue changing for the better, one day you will wake up and you will be used to it. You will realize that keeping yourself healthy is not a challenge anymore, but a regular part of your system.

ABOUT THE AUTHOR

Stacia G. Browne has always had a keen interest in the juicing process. Her mother used to juice all the time, but Stacia always opted not to have what was prepared. It was when she became older that she had a greater appreciation for the benefits that juicing had for the body.

When she started to gain a lot of excess weight, she started to juice and found that she was not only losing the excess weight that she had gained, but that she had a lot of energy to get her through her daily tasks. Her main aim was to spread the benefits of juicing to as many persons as she could as it was a much healthier lifestyle.